Natural Remedies
for Health, Beauty and
Home

Baking Soda

Josephine Simon

Copyrights

Disclaimer and Terms of Use

ISBN: 978-1537654096

Printed in the United States

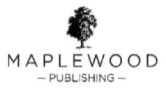

MAPLEWOOD
– PUBLISHING –

Contents

Introduction

Who would have known that that box of white powder in your kitchen would be a cheap but amazing ingredient for health, beauty, cleaning, and other surprising uses?

I used to know baking soda only as that intriguing ingredient in making cookies. I had no idea what it was for. All the other ingredients in baking were somewhat self-explanatory – sugar for sweetening, vanilla for flavor, flour to give structure, chocolate to make everything yummier (of course), but what was this mysterious powder called baking soda?

Baking soda is known by other names such as *cooking soda*, *bread soda*, *sodium bicarbonate*, *bicarbonate of soda*, *sodium acid carbonate* or *sodium hydrogen carbonate*. Its scientific formula is $NaHCO_3$.

From spiritual cleansing agent to yeast substitute

It's interesting to note that the ancient Egyptians used *natron*, a natural mineral found in springs and salt lakes. Natron is a hydrated form of baking soda. To the Egyptians, natron was highly-prized because of its many significant uses. Egyptians found a way to convert it into a dye for making hieroglyphics.

It was also the ultimate cleanser. Natron was used for household cleaning purposes, deodorizing, and even for pest control. It had cosmetic uses as well – cleansing the skin and teeth. Most significantly, it was used for mummification. Natron was used to preserve the body of the departed as wholly as possible. In ancient Egyptian culture, beauty and physical wholeness were all tied to spirituality. Natron served the function of physical as well as spiritual cleansing.

In 1791, a French doctor and chemist named Nicholas LeBlanc discovered a way to make soda ash. Soda ash was in high demand at the time for industrial purposes, such as soap-making, but the natural sources were limited. LeBlanc's process of making soda ash also produced sodium bicarbonate as an intermediate product. At that time, it was called *saleratus.* In colonial America, saleratus was also known to have leavening properties, though not of consistent quality. Literature of that period mention its use as a fish preservative.

In 1843, an English chemist named Alfred Bird discovered that he could combine baking soda with corn flour and cream of tartar to make a substitute for yeast, to which his wife was allergic. His discovery paved the way for the shift from dense yeast-based breads to light and more conveniently made cakes.

From England, baking soda was introduced to the United States. And, in 1946, Austin Church and John Dwight started a baking soda manufacturing plant in New York. The well-known Arm & Hammer brand was established by Church's son, John.

Nowadays, many baking soda brands promote their product as coming from a natural source. This natural source is known now as *trona,* which is also actually natron. The state of Wyoming is one of the world's leading sources of trona. Trona figures significantly in the US economy as it is also used in the manufacture of important materials such as glass, soaps, detergents, and paper.

The many uses of baking soda – not just a leavening agent

The use of baking soda, it is said, came full circle in the year 2000, when school children learned to use it to mummify hotdogs. We have come a long way from the time of the ancient Egyptians who used baking soda in its natural form as a spiritual, holistic agent for cleansing, preserving, healing, and beautifying. But, as you see in the list below, baking soda it still used similarly today. Known for some time only as a baking ingredient for leavening, baking soda now proves to be useful in other ways (though some of these uses were already known thousands of years earlier by the ancient Egyptians).

For cleaning
Baking soda is a mild and natural cleaner for pots, copper, the teeth, skin, hair, batteries, floors, tiles, sinks, clothes, and so much more. Even without any strong perfumes, it removes undesirable odors and leaves everything smelling clean.

For beauty
Baking soda can make skin softer and smoother, hair shinier, and teeth whiter. It definitely can help you become more beautiful.

For health
As a mild alkali, baking soda can help combat diseases or health conditions related to too much acidity like arthritis, skin problems, acid reflux, and even cancer.

For gardening
Baking soda can keep bugs away, act as fertilizer, kill weeds, and help you in your yard and garden in many ways.

For sports
Athletes use baking soda to improve their performance and endurance. Baking soda can also minimize any pain, injuries, or exhaustion from physical exertion.

For pets
The benefits from baking soda are not just limited to us humans. Your pets can benefit from all its wonderful properties as well – for cleaning, deodorizing, and repelling insects.

As you skim through this book, you'll discover many surprising but highly effective uses for baking soda.

Health benefits

In our modern world, with today's modern lifestyle, we are bombarded with factors that make us more susceptible to disease. Pollution, stress, chemical exposure, lack of exercise, and a diet rich in refined sugars, preservatives, fat, meat, alcohol, and caffeine all produce too much acidity in the body. To restore the body's acid-alkali or pH balance, alkaline salts in the body will be directed towards the bloodstream, leading to depletion in other organs. For example, meat is acidic in the body. Too much of it will cause an imbalance. To correct this, the body may turn to calcium reserves in the skeletal system to restore the blood's normal pH level. This could result in diseases related to the skeletal system such as osteoporosis or bone loss. Additionally, viruses, bacteria, and fungi all thrive in acidic surroundings but are effectively deterred in an alkaline environment. Other diseases resulting from too much acidity in the body are fatigue, acid reflux, heartburn, stomach upset, arthritis, muscle pain, and a host of diseases or a general weakening of the immune system. The most alarming fact in connection with body acidity is that it is the breeding ground for cancer. Incredibly, this fact was already known in 1931, when Dr. Otto Warburg revealed his findings on this. He even won the Nobel Peace Prize for his findings. And yet it is still relatively unknown to many.

Disease-causing microorganisms refuse to grow in an alkaline environment. By keeping our bodies alkaline, we can avoid many ailments. Baking soda has been found to effectively maintain alkalinity in the body. More than a century ago, the US Pharmacopoeia recognized the efficacy of baking soda in neutralizing stomach acids. It was used to ease symptoms of many problems with stomach acidity and indigestion. In 2009, a study published in the Journal of the American Society of Nephrology showed that using baking soda effectively arrested the progression of kidney disease in 134 patients. Baking soda also eases the symptoms of a cold or flu and can even stop it on its tracks. It can curb cravings for cigarettes and sweets.

Because baking soda so effectively makes our body more alkaline, it has been found to be a safe, natural, and cheap remedy for such conditions as stomach acidity, gout, acid reflux, kidney disease, skin irritations, body odor, and cancer. It helps protect the body from the negative side effects of chemotherapy and radiation therapy for cancer. You will find many helpful and effective recipes in this book that will help you overcome many ailments, boost your immunity and prevent onset of disease.

Safety

Baking soda is natural and non-toxic. However, as with everything else, it is always best to exercise caution. It should not be used beyond what is recommended as this could upset the body's natural pH balance. Some special precautions should be noted.

Vegetarian and Vegans
People who consume a lot of vegetables and fruit may not need to balance their pH, or may only be slightly acidic. So their consumption of baking soda may have to be less than the recommended dosages.

Restrictions
Although the form of sodium in baking soda does not react in the body the same way that sodium in table salt does (it is the interaction of sodium and chloride that is said to influence hypertension), it is best to exercise caution. Consumption of large amounts of sodium could raise blood pressure, cause swelling or edema, lower potassium levels, and aggravate heart or kidney diseases. Pregnant women are prone to edema and therefore should not use baking soda internally. Normally, it is recommended that one should NOT consume more than 4 teaspoons of baking soda per day. Persons taking prescription drugs should consult their doctors before taking baking soda internally.

Allergic Reactions
Some people may have hypersensitive or allergic reactions to baking soda. Though rare, allergic reactions such as stinging and burning sensation on the skin, hives, rashes, wheezing, swelling, and anaphylactic

shock are possible. If any of the mentioned symptoms is experienced, discontinue use immediately and see a doctor.

Skin and Hair Damage
Constant use without monitoring pH could cause external irritation, drying, and breaking of the skin and hair.

Sensitivity
Individuals with sensitivity to baking soda may have external reactions like skin irritation or internal reactions like nausea, muscle spasms, dizziness, or vomiting.

Low Potassium Level
If you have a tendency to have a low potassium level in your blood, baking soda may lower it even further.

Alkaline Burn
Do not consume baking soda purely on its own or in concentrated form. Too much or very strong alkalinity can cause burns the same way strong acids do.

pH strip or indicators
The use of pH paper is advisable in order to have a better basis for adjusting one's pH using baking soda. pH can be measured through one's saliva or urine. Keep in mind that pH can vary depending on food intake, stress, activity, and other factors, so it is best to note one's pH 4-5 times a day. Get your average pH, and adjust your baking soda intake accordingly. Ideally, urine's pH should range from 6.5 to 7. Keep your drinking water at pH 7.2 to 7.5.

Aluminum

Some baking soda brands have "aluminum-free" stated in their packaging. This has caused some confusion as to the safety of conventional baking soda versus those taken directly from the natural source or from *trona*. Although baking soda can be produced chemically using the *Solvay process,* there is no aluminum involved. However, most proponents of the use of baking soda still recommend those sourced naturally, especially if it is to be taken internally.

Recipes for Health

Basic Body Alkalizer/Cold & Flu Remedy

You'll need:
1/4 teaspoon baking soda
1/2 glass water

Instructions:
1. Dissolve the baking soda in water.
2. Take on an empty stomach upon waking and before going to bed.
3. Take at the onset of cold and flu symptoms.

Body Alkalizer I (to alkalize blood)

You'll need:
1/4-1/3 teaspoon baking soda
12-16 ounces water (tap or bottled)

Instructions:
1. Dissolve the baking soda in water.
2. Drink 1 glass in the morning and 1 in the evening, swishing in the mouth before swallowing.
3. Drink an extra glass for heartburn.

Alkalizer II

You'll need:
3/4-1teaspoon baking soda
1 gallon distilled or reverse-osmosis water
OR
1/2 teaspoon baking soda
1 gallon tap or bottled water

Instructions:
1. Dissolve the baking soda in water.
2. Drink 1 glass in the morning and 1 in the evening, swishing in the mouth before swallowing.
3. Drink an extra glass for heartburn.

Alkalizer III (to reduce stomach acid and acidosis)

You'll need:
1/2 teaspoon baking powder
2 tablespoons freshly-squeezed lemon juice or apple cider vinegar
1 cup water (8 ounces)

Instructions:
1. First, add the lemon juice/vinegar to baking soda.
2. Allow to fizz.
3. When fizzing has stopped, add water and mix.
4. Drink in one sitting.

Cold and Flu Treatment

You'll need:
1/2 teaspoon baking powder
1 cup cool water

Instructions:
1. 1st day
   Take 6 doses at 2 hour intervals.
2. 2nd day
   Take 4 doses at 2 hour intervals.
3. 3rd day
   Take once in the morning and once in the evening.
4. Succeeding days
   Take once in the morning until symptoms subside.

Alkaline Supplement for Cancer Patients

You'll need:
2 teaspoons baking soda (12 grams)
2 cups water
Any low-calorie sweetener of choice (optional)

Instructions:
1. Whisk ingredients together.
2. Sip over the course of 1 or 2 hours.
3. Repeat 3 times a day.

Heartburn or Indigestion Remedy

You'll need:
1/2 teaspoon baking soda
1/2 cup water

Instructions:
1. Dissolve the baking soda in water.
2. Drink 1 or 2 hours after meals.

NOTE: Should be used as first aid only and not repeatedly. See doctor for persistent symptoms of heartburn.

Soothing Bath (for psoriasis and itchiness)

You'll need:
1/2 cup baking soda
Tub of bathwater

Instructions:
1. Dissolve baking soda in bathwater.
2. Allow skin to air-dry after bathing.

Soothing Skin Paste (for sunburn, insect bites, allergic rashes, ivy rash, and pimples)

You'll need:
Baking soda
Water

Instructions:
1. Mix together to make a paste and apply on affected area.
2. Leave on as long as tolerated.
3. For pimples, leave on overnight.
4. Rinse off.

Basic Toothpaste

You'll need:
Baking soda
Water

Instructions:
1. Dip you toothbrush in water and shake off any excess.
2. Dip your toothbrush in baking soda.
3. Brush teeth as you normally do.

NOTE: Use only once a week. Baking soda's abrasive quality may destroy tooth enamel.

Anti-cavity and Whitening Toothpaste

You'll need:
1/4 cup coconut oil (softened or in liquid state)
1 1/2 tablespoons baking soda
1 packet stevia powder (or to taste)
Mint essential oil or cinnamon oil (according to desired taste), food grade

Instructions:
1. Combine ingredients thoroughly.
2. Use small spoon, spatula, or popsicle stick to apply a small amount on toothbrush.
3. Use like regular toothpaste.

Antiseptic Tooth and Gum Paste

You'll need:
1 tablespoon sea salt
6 tablespoons baking soda

Instructions:
1. Place in a blender to make a paste.
2. Wet the tip of your index finger and dip into paste.
3. Rub on gums and teeth and spit out any excess.
4. Leave on for about 5-15 minutes.
5. Rinse thoroughly with water.

Toothache Rinse

You'll need:
1 tablespoon Baking Soda
1/2 cup water
1/8 teaspoon salt

Instructions:
1. Mix together.
2. Swish around affected area.

NOTE: High in sodium. Do not swallow. Rinse mouth thoroughly after use.

Natural Mouthwash (to fight bad breath, canker sores, and other mouth infections)

You'll need:
1/2 teaspoon baking soda
8 ounces water
1/8 teaspoon table salt
A few drops mint oil or flavor (or any oil of desired flavor), food grade

Instructions:
1. Combine ingredients, and store in a bottle.
2. Swish in mouth for 30 seconds to 1 minute after meals or as needed.

Razor Burn Soother (Mild antiseptic and anti-inflammatory)

You'll need:
1 tablespoon baking soda
1 cup water

Instructions:
1. Mix well.
2. Moisten a cotton ball with this solution.
3. Apply on affected area and hold for about 1minute.
4. Rinse with cold water.

Hand-Cleaning Powder

You'll need:
1 cup baking soda
15-20 drops tea tree oil

Instructions:
1. Mix together or shake in a jar.
2. Place in a container with perforations like a salt shaker.
3. Shake a small amount on damp hands.
4. Rub hands together gently.
5. Rinse thoroughly.

Toenail Fungus Foot Soak (also Athlete's Foot Remedy)

You'll need:
4 tablespoons baking soda
1 cup apple cider vinegar
Water (to soak feet in)

Instructions:
1. Prepare two basins for your foot soak.
2. Fill both basins with just enough water for soaking your feet.
3. In the first basin, mix in the vinegar.
4. In the second basin, dissolve the baking soda.
5. Soak your feet or the affected foot in the vinegar soak for 15 minutes.
6. Pat dry with paper towels.
7. Next, soak in baking soda bath for 15 minutes. Pat dry.
8. Do this twice a day.

Treatment for Splinters

You'll need:
1 tablespoon baking soda
3/4 cup water

Instructions:
1. Soak affected area in solution twice a day.
2. Splinter should come out on its own after 2-3 days of soaking.

Remedies for Dandruff

Basic Paste

You'll need:
1-2 teaspoons baking soda
Water

Instructions:
1. Gradually add a few drops of water to baking soda to make until a paste is formed.
2. Apple on scalp with fingers, massaging gently for 2 minutes.
3. Rinse thoroughly with cool water.
4. Do not use shampoo after treatment.

Baking Soda and Lemon Juice

You'll need:
1-2 teaspoons baking soda
About 1 teaspoon freshly-squeezed lemon juice

Instructions:
1. Gradually add lemon juice by drops into baking soda to make a paste (more or less juice will be needed to achieve desire consistency).
2. Massage paste over scalp for 2 minutes.
3. Leave on for 5 minutes.
4. Rinse thoroughly with cool water.
5. Do this twice a week to control dandruff.

Baking Soda-Apple Cider Vinegar Paste

You'll need:
2 teaspoons baking soda
Apple cider vinegar

Instructions:
1. Combine to make a paste.
2. Apply on scalp, scrubbing gently to loosen dandruff.
3. Rinse thoroughly with cool water.
4. Repeat twice a week.

Baking Soda and Ginger Paste

You'll need:
1 teaspoon baking soda
1 teaspoon fresh ginger juice
A few drops water

Instructions:
1. Mix baking soda, ginger juice, and a few drops water together to make a paste.
2. Massage into scalp.
3. Leave on for 1-2 minutes.
4. Rinse with cool water.
5. Do this once a week.

Holy Basil Hair Pack

You'll need:

1/2 cup fresh holy basil
1 teaspoon baking soda

Instructions:

1. Wash the holy basil and drain.
2. Puree in a blender to make a paste.
3. Add baking soda and mix well.
4. Apply on hair and scalp as a pack.
5. Leave on to dry for a few minutes.
6. Rinse thoroughly with cool water.

Saline Solution for Sinus Irrigation I

You'll need:
1 cup water, heated to desired warmth
1 teaspoon sea salt
1/8 teaspoon baking soda

Instructions:
1. Place salt and baking soda into neti pot or saline spray bottle.
2. Add the warm water.
3. Shake to mix.
4. Follow the directions in your container for irrigating/spraying your nasal passages.

Saline Solution II (stronger, for acute sinusitis and severely clogged nose)

You'll need:
1 quart water
3 teaspoons salt
1 teaspoon baking soda

Instructions:
1. Mix ingredients in a microwavable container.
2. Microwave to heat and dissolve.
3. Allow to cool down.
4. When temperature is tolerable or lukewarm, place in saline spray bottle or neti pot and use according to container's instructions.

Earwax Softener

You'll need:
1/2 teaspoon baking soda
2 ounces water

Instructions:
1. Dissolve baking soda in water and place in dropper bottle.
2. Drop into ears at least once a day for 3 to 14 days.

NOTE: Not recommended for people who have perforated eardrums. If pain is severe and there is unusual drainage from the ear, see a doctor.

Scab Softener and Remover

You'll need:
2 tablespoons baking soda
1/2 cup water

Instructions:
1. Mix together to make a paste.
2. Apply on scab and leave on for 15 minutes.
3. Rinse off.

Mild antiseptic for scar prevention

You'll need:
1 teaspoon baking soda
1/2 cup water

Instructions:
1. Dissolve baking soda in water.
2. Soak gauze with solution and apply to the skin just after scab has come off.
3. Cover with bandage.
4. Leave uncovered at least 12 hours a day.

Gargle for Sore Throat

You'll need:
1/2 teaspoon baking soda
1 cup warm water

Instructions:
1. Dissolve baking soda in water.
2. Gargle to soothe inflammation.

Recipes for Beauty and Personal Care

Fizzy Aromatherapy Tablets

You'll need:

1 cup baking soda
1/2 cup citric acid
1/2 cup cornstarch
10 drops orange essential oil
10 drops lavender essential oil
10 drops lemongrass essential oil

Instructions:

1. In a small mixing bowl, mix together the baking soda, citric acid, and cornstarch until lump-free.
2. Gradually mix in essential oils.
3. Spritz with water and stir. Continue spritzing and stirring until sand-like in consistency.
4. Fill silicon molds, packing well. Allow to dry (about 8 hours).
5. Remove from molds carefully.
6. For shower: Place one at the bottom of your shower. It will fizz and release the scent as water from the shower falls on it.
7. For tub: Add to bath water. The scents will energize and refresh.

Facial Cleanser and Exfoliant

You'll need:
3/4 teaspoon baking soda
1/4 teaspoon water

Instructions:
1. Make a paste with baking soda and water.
2. Gently massage over face in circular motion.

NOTE: Do not use with other acne products.

Strawberry and Baking Soda Whitening Toothpaste

You'll need:
1/2 teaspoon baking soda
1 ripe strawberry, cleaned

Instructions:
1. Crush the strawberry and baking soda to make a coarse paste.
2. Use index finger to spread over teeth.
3. Leave on for 5 minutes.
4. Brush teeth and rinse well.

NOTE: Do this only once a week to avoid destroying natural tooth enamel.

Hair Shampoo (to remove chlorine build-up)

You'll need:
1/2 teaspoon baking soda
1 pint water

Instructions:
1. Apply to hair.
2. Rinse thoroughly.

Dry Shampoo

You'll need:
1 teaspoon baking soda
1 teaspoon cocoa powder (if you have dark hair)

Instructions:
1. Distribute around hair roots.
2. Brush off.

Hair Shampoo (to remove hair product residue)

You'll need:
1 1/2 tablespoons shampoo (any of your choice)
1/2 teaspoon baking soda

Instructions:
1. Mix together and shampoo as usual.

Body Scrub and Cleanser

You'll need:
1 cup baking soda
Filtered water
5 drops essential oil of choice (like lavender, vanilla, orange, lemon, peppermint, vanilla)

Instructions:
1. In a bowl, drop the essential oil gradually while mixing the baking powder.
2. When oil is evenly incorporated into baking soda, add water gradually by the spoonful to make a paste.
3. Store in a wide-mouthed jar or container.
4. Scoop out with hands and rub on skin.
5. Rinse with water.
6. No need to soap body after use.

Baking Soda and Oatmeal Soap (soothing; for dry, irritated, or sensitive skin)

You'll need:
16 ounces baking soda
3.2 ounces distilled water
16 ounces grated Castile rebatch (soap base), cured
0.2 ounce oat extract
0.5 ounce colloidal oatmeal
0.2 ounce rolled oats
Loaf pan or wood loaf mold, with silicon liner or other silicon mold

Instructions:
1. Combine baking soda and distilled water. Stir with a spoon.
2. Place grated Castile in double boiler over medium heat.
3. Add baking soda mixture to grated Castile in double boiler. Stir with silicon spoon.
4. Add colloidal mixture and stir.
5. The grated Castile should be melting into a paste. Turn up heat, if needed.
6. Add oat extract. Continue stirring.
7. After about 20 minutes over double boiler, melted Castile rebatch should have thick, sticky, and oatmeal-like texture. Add drops amounts of water if consistency is more clay-like or too dry. Be careful not to add too much water or else you will have a soft soap that is difficult to mold.
8. When texture has reached mashed potato-like consistency, it is ready to be put in molds.
9. Scoop into molds.

10. Lift the mold slightly off the table and drop gently to remove any air bubbles. Do this a few times.
11. Sprinkle rolled oats on top for decorative finish.
12. Let sit for 2-4 days.
13. Unmold carefully and cut into bars.

Soaking Solution for dentures

You'll need:
1 teaspoon baking soda
Water (enough to cover dentures)
1 teaspoon white vinegar (optional)

Instructions:
1. Dissolve baking soda in water.
2. Add vinegar.
3. Soak dentures for a few hours or overnight.
4. Brush clean and rinse.

Basic Natural Deodorant

You'll need:
Baking soda
Water

Instructions:
1. Mix together to make a milk-like liquid.
2. Rub on feet and underarms.

Baking Soda and Coconut Oil Deodorant

You'll need:
2 tablespoons baking soda
1/3 cup arrowroot powder
1/3 cup coconut oil
A few drops essential oil of choice like mint, lavender, or cinnamon (optional)

Instructions:
1. Mix the baking soda and arrowroot powder together.
2. Gradually add to coconut oil while stirring. Smooth out any lumps and continue mixing until creamy or deodorant-like in consistency. Note: Coconut oil is liquid in warm temperature.
3. Add in essential oil and mix well (optional).
4. Use fingers to apply a small amount on clean armpits. Start with the size of half a pea, increase if needed until you've determined the right amount for you.
5. Let dry for about 2 minutes before dressing.

Pampering Foot Spa and Callus Softener

You'll need:
For soaking/softening calluses
2 tablespoons baking soda
Warm water for soaking feet
A few drops essential oil of choice (lavender, mint, lemon, vanilla, etc.)

Scrub
1 tablespoon baking soda
1 teaspoon brown sugar
1 teaspoon water

Lotion or moisturizer
Warm towel or foot wrap

Instructions:
1. Combine ingredients for soaking in a foot basin.
2. Soak feet for about 15 minutes.
3. Combine ingredients for scrub in a bowl.
4. Spread all over feet, massage and scrub to remove hardened skin.
5. Rinse and pat dry.
6. Massage generous amount of lotion or moisturizer.
7. Wrap feet with warm towel.
8. Let sit for 5-10 minutes.

Gentle Baking Soda and Honey Facewash (antifungal and anti-acne)

You'll need:
1 teaspoon baking powder
1 tablespoon honey

Instructions:
1. Combine together in the palm of your hand.
2. Apply on face, massaging in circular motion.
3. Leave on for 1 minute.
4. Rinse with warm water.

Nail Whitener

You'll need:
2 teaspoons baking soda
1 teaspoon hydrogen peroxide

Instructions:
1. Combine ingredients.
2. Apply on nails with a toothbrush or nail brush.
3. Let sit for 3-5 minutes.
4. Rinse thoroughly.
5. Moisturize hands after treatment.

Artificial Tan Eraser

You'll need:
2 teaspoons baking soda
1 teaspoon freshly squeezed lemon juice

Instructions:
1. Mix together.
2. Rub over area to be "erased."
3. Wipe off, if needed.

Makeup Brush Cleaner

You'll need:
2 teaspoons baking soda
1 cup warm water

Instructions:
1. Dip brushes in solution.
2. Rinse thoroughly.
3. Pat dry with paper towels.
4. Allow to air dry thoroughly before use.

Bath Salts for Soothing Soak (also Foot Bath)

You'll need:
4 teaspoons baking soda
1 cup sea salt
1 cup Epsom salt
8-10 drops essential oil of choice
    Possible choices:
        Lavender –calming
        Orange/lemon – energizing, refreshing
        Peppermint – refreshing
        Frankincense – skin toning, calming
        Eucalyptus- invigorating
        Vanilla- calming

Instructions:
1. Mix ingredients thoroughly.
2. Store in airtight glass jar.
3. Add 1 cup to bath water, 1/2 cup to basin of warm water for foot soak.

Baking Soda and Citrus Brightening Face Mask

You'll need:
1 tablespoon baking soda
1 tablespoon freshly squeezed, strained orange, lemon, or grapefruit juice

Instructions:
1. Combine and massage over cleansed face.
2. Leave on for 20 minutes. NOTE: Some people are sensitive to this combination. Rinse off immediately if you experience a stinging or burning sensation.
3. Rinse thoroughly and pat dry.
4. Moisturize face.

Recipes for Household Use

DIY All-Around cleaner

You'll need:

1 cup baking soda

Essential oils (like mint, lemon, or lavender)

3 tablespoons white vinegar

Instructions:

1. Combine together baking soda and oils and store in airtight container.
2. Sprinkle over surface to be cleaned.
3. Drizzle with vinegar (optional).
4. Scrub or wipe with a sponge or rag.
5. Rinse well.

Cleaner for Pots and Pans

You'll need:

Baking soda (to cover grease and grime in pots)

Instructions:

1. Soak in baking soda for 15-20 minutes.
2. Scrub off baking soda.
3. Rinse.

Dry Carpet Cleaner

You'll need:

Baking soda (enough to cover carpet in a fine coat)

Instructions:
1. Sprinkle carpet with baking soda.
2. Scrub stubborn dirt.
3. Let soak for 15-20 minutes.
4. Vacuum off.

Microwave Cleaner

You'll need:

1 teaspoon baking soda

Instructions:
1. Sprinkle baking soda on dry rag.
2. Wipe grease and dirt off microwave with this.
3. Wipe again with wet rag, if needed.

Drain Cleaner

You'll need:
1 cup baking soda
1 cup apple cider vinegar
Hot water

Instructions:
1. Dump baking soda into drain followed by vinegar.
2. Let bubble and soak for 15 minutes.
3. Rinse with hot water.
4. You may use more or less or the mixture, depending on the severity of clogging.

Dish Degreaser

You'll need:
1 teaspoon baking soda
1/2 cup dishwashing detergent

Instructions:
1. Mix baking soda with detergent for extra degreasing power or add to regular dishwashing cycle.
2. For stubborn grease, sprinkle baking soda over dishes and scrub with sponge before regular dishwashing.

Grease Fire Extinguisher

You'll need:
2 cups baking soda (or more depending on size of flame)

Instructions:
1. If possible and safe, turn off gas or electricity first.
2. Pour the baking soda over the flames to immediately extinguish small and minor grease fires.
3. For stove top fires or camp fires, stand at a distance and throw cups full towards the flames.
4. Call the fire department for large fires.

Coffee and Tea Pot/Cup Stain Remover

You'll need:
1/4 cup baking soda
1 quart warm water

Instructions:
1. Fill pot or cup with solution for a few hours to remove tough stains.
2. Scrub and rinse off.

Fabric Softener

You'll need:
1/2 cup baking soda per rinse load

Instructions:
1. Add baking soda to final rinse cycle.

Detergent Booster

You'll need:
1/2 cup baking powder

Instructions:
1. Add to wash cycle along with detergent. This helps soften hard water, reduce suds, remove laundry odors, and stabilize water pH for better detergent and bleach action.

Iron Cleaner

You'll need:
Baking soda
Water
White vinegar

Instructions:
1. With baking soda and water, make a paste.
2. Apply on a white cloth.
3. Scrub bottom of iron to remove build up.
4. Wipe clean with cloth dipped in white vinegar.

Bed Bug Killer

You'll need:
Baking soda (a lot, about 10 boxes)

Instructions:
1. Vacuum floor, chairs, furniture, beddings, and anywhere you suspect there may be bed bugs.
2. Dust mattresses generously with baking soda, taking special attention to edges, before covering with plastic mattress cover (recommended), or sheets.
3. Dust tops of sheets with baking soda in a thin film.
4. Dust other places with bed bugs.
5. Spread baking soda over floor and use a broom to spread and to fill crevices. Leave on floor.
6. Repeat procedure frequently.
7. Treatment may take a whole year before bed bugs are under control or totally exterminated.

Cleaning Solution for Brushes and Combs

You'll need:
2 teaspoons baking soda
1 cup water

Instructions:
1. Apply solution to combs and brushes.
2. For extra grimy brushes and combs, soak for 2 hours and scrub.
3. Rinse thoroughly.

All-Around Deodorizer

You'll need:
Baking soda (quantity depends on need and object to be deodorized)

Instructions:
For shoes, lunchboxes, trashcans, stuffed toys, and car seats:
1. To deodorize, sprinkle on or inside the object, let sit for 15 minutes, and shake clean or vacuum.

For refrigerators and closets:
1. Place an opened box on a shelf at the back of the refrigerator or closet.

For cutting boards:
1. Scrub with baking soda and rinse well.

Perfectly Safe Bug Killer

You'll need:

1 cup baking soda

1 cup finely powdered sugar

Instructions:

1. Combine ingredients thoroughly. Sugar should be very fine so that ant will can't tell it apart from the soda.
2. Sprinkle on infested areas. After ingesting the powder, the soda will aerate inside them and kill crawling insects. Especially effective on ants and roaches.

Diaper Soak to Remove Urine Smell

You'll need:
1/2 cup baking soda

Instructions:
1. Add 1/2 cup to diapers soaked in water.
2. Agitate for 2 minutes.
3. Let soak overnight.
4. Drain and launder as usual.

Recipes for Garden Use

Cabbage Worm Killer

You'll need:

1 cup flour

1 cup baking soda

Instructions:

1. Mix together thoroughly.
2. Dust on leaves. Cabbage worms will eat this together with the leaves and die in a day or two.

Gnats and Fungus Spray

You'll need:

4 teaspoons baking soda

1 teaspoon biodegradable soap

1 gallon water

Instructions:

1. Combine all ingredients thoroughly.
2. Spray soil where there are gnats, and spray leaves that have a fungus as needed.

Natural Fungicide for Grapes and Roses

You'll need:
4 teaspoons baking soda
1 gallon water

Instructions:
1. Combine well.
2. Spray over black fungus in roses.
3. It is time to spray grapes and vines when fruits begin to appear.

Mildew Spray

You'll need:
1 tablespoon baking soda
1 gallon water
1 tablespoon vegetable oil
1 tablespoon dishwashing liquid

Instructions:
1. Combine all ingredients.
2. Spray once a week on impatiens, zinnias, lilacs, squash, and cucumbers.
3. After spraying, remove from direct sunlight to prevent leaf burn.

Weed Killer

You'll need:

Baking soda (to cover areas that need weeding)

Instructions:

1. Sweep or dust areas like sidewalks, cracks in driveway, or patios generously with baking soda to discourage weed growth and kill sprouting weeds.

Crab Grass Killer

You'll need:

Baking soda
Water

Instructions:

1. Wet unwanted crabgrass with water.
2. Dust generously with baking soda. The crabgrass should die in 2-3 days. Be careful not to get baking soda on lawn grass.

Recipes for Pets

Deodorizer for Kitty Litter

You'll need:

1 or 2 cups baking soda

Instructions:

1. Cover bottom of kitty litter box with baking soda.
2. Add kitty litter as usual.

Pet Bedding Deodorizer

You'll need:

Baking soda (enough to cover pet beddings)

Instructions:

1. Sprinkle over both sides of beddings.
2. Let sit for at least 15 minutes. Scrub particularly moist or smelly areas.
3. Vacuum.

Skunk Stink Deodorizer

You'll need:

1 quart of 3% hydrogen peroxide
1/4 cup baking soda
1 teaspoon liquid soap

Instructions:

1. Combine well.
2. Bathe infected animal with solution.
3. Rinse well and dry.
4. Discard unused solution.

Pet "Accident" Remover

You'll need:

Club soda
Baking soda

Instructions:

1. Scrub the "accident" with club soda and let dry.
2. Sprinkle generously with baking soda.
3. Let stand.
4. Vacuum.

Antiseptic for Minor Paw Cuts

You'll need:
Baking soda

Instructions:
1. Dip the affected part in baking soda.
2. Press down on cut to arrest bleeding. This is especially helpful for nail-trimming accidents.

Aquarium Water Conditioner

You'll need:
1 tablespoon baking soda
1 cup dechlorinated water

Instructions:
1. Add very gradually to fish tank water, over the course of 2 hours.
2. This helps maintain proper pH of water.

Recipes for Other Uses

Septic Care

You'll need:
1 cup baking soda for each drain

Instructions:
1. Pour 1 cup into drain once a week to keep water flowing freely and pH of septic tank at desirable level.

Fruit and Vegetable Cleaner

You'll need:
1 teaspoon
1/2 cup water

Instructions:
1. Moisten clean sponge with solution and scrub fruit and vegetables.
2. Rinse well.
3. For thin-skinned fruits and vegetables, simply swish the liquid over the surface or soak for 5 minutes and rinse.

Car Cleaner

You'll need:
1/4 cup baking soda
1 cup warm water

Instructions:
1. Make a paste and use to clean car. Can be used for seats, window, lights, windows, and more.
2. To make non-abrasive, dilute into a gallon of water and use to wipe car.
3. Rinse off.

Sports Drink I

You'll need:
1 quart water
1/2 teaspoon baking soda
1/2 teaspoon salt
1/4 teaspoon potassium-based salt substitute
2 tablespoons sugar
1-2 teaspoons lemon juice or according to taste (optional)
Honey, to taste (optional)

Instructions:
1. Combine all ingredients thoroughly or place in a bottle and shake vigorously.

Sports Drink II

You'll need:
1/2 teaspoon salt
1/4 teaspoon baking soda
7 cups water
1/2 cup lemon or orange juice
1 tablespoon lime juice
1/2 teaspoon honey (for athletes) OR 1/4 teaspoon liquid stevia (if ill)

Instructions:
1. Dissolve salt and baking soda in water.
2. Add juices and mix well.
3. Add honey gradually by stirring until dissolved.
4. Keeps for 1 week in refrigerator.

Conclusion

To have something so natural and so helpful yet so cheap is a rare thing nowadays.

How refreshing to know that that this simple white powder that you use for baking actually has a myriad of uses! Most importantly, it could be the key to wellness without having to spend a fortune.

Try out the recipes! You have nothing to lose! Many have already tested these recipes and swear by them. By using baking soda, you contribute to making a healthier, cleaner, more natural, and safer world.

More Books from Josephine Simon

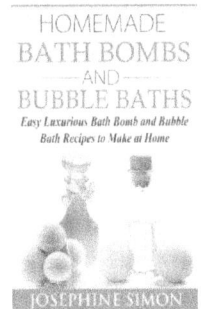 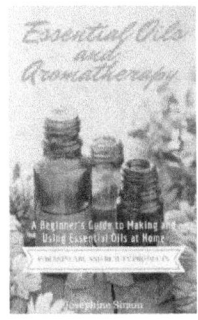 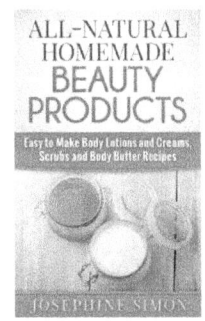

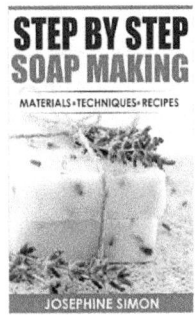 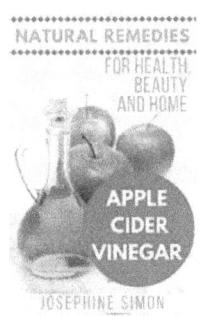 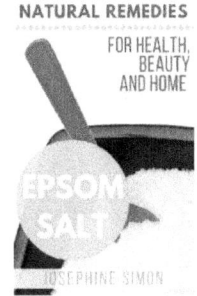

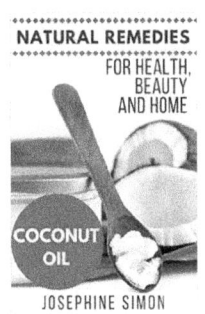

www.ingramcontent.com/pod-product-compliance
Lightning Source LLC
Chambersburg PA
CBHW060218290526
45789CB00003B/1313